REPAIR

YOUR

GUT HEALTH

Steps, Habits and Recipes to Help You Transform Your Gut, Mental and Physical Health In 28 Days

ROSALINE SEA

REPAIR YOUR GUT HEALTH

Copyright © 2024 by Rosaline Sea

Acknowledgments

Thank you to Late Mr. Thaddeus J.O.A. I miss you everyday.

TABLE OF CONTENT

INTRODUCTION..**4**

CHAPTER ONE..**8**
Knowing About Your Gut Health....................................8
The Gut-Brain Connection..10
The Digestive System..12
Indications That Your Gut health Is Bad.........................22

CHAPTER TWO..**31**
Repair Your Gut Health..31
Simple Steps to Repair Your Gut Permanently:...................31
The Elimination Stage...32
The top ten foods that are detrimental to gut health include but not limited to;....................................33
Additionally, routines, and habits, such as these, can also affect your gut health:................................36
The Repair Stage..46
Gut Health Healing Foods..47
Lifestyle Changes...66
The Re-introduction Stage.......................................88
The Maintenance Stage...90

CHAPTER THREE..**96**
Food recipes that support good gut health.......................96
Breakfast Recipes...97
Lunch Recipes..114
Dinner Recipes...124

Smoothie Recipes.. 147
Tea Recipes... 152

Conclusions... 163

INTRODUCTION

I do not remember a time when I was not bloated. Well, not until 18 months ago. I also do not remember a time when I didn't have abdominal pain, I was always in constant pain.

When I was in the university, I had roommates and anytime I had to use the toilet, they would all leave the room because of how bad my poop smelt, as a matter of fact, I spent more time alone than I did with people because I always had a need to fart, and my farts smelled terrible.

Out of concern for me, one day, one of my roommates asked me how frequently I used the toilet. I casually told her; 'Once a week' as sometimes I could go up to 10 days without feeling pressured to use the toilet, or even if I did, I would not be able to pass anything out, which I later found out was responsible for why my poop used to smell so badly.

I could tell she was very worried when she replied that it wasn't okay, as she usually goes at least once a day.

I did not know at the time that this was also the reason for why I was always tired, I could not stand for more than 5 minutes without needing to sit on a chair, I was only 20 years old at the time, and I always felt dizzy after doing a few chores, not to mention the frequent bouts of sadness and mood swings I had, pale skin, and of course, really bad acne I experienced, I did not know how bad I had it with my gut health, and this went on for years.

I turned 25 years old, some 18 months ago, and like most people when they turn a new age, have new resolutions and I resolved to hit the gym and get in shape, and this included learning about food and exercise and my entire well being in general.

With my new resolution came all forms of new information and I finally discovered that my gut health was suffering, and has been for years.

It took the 6 months to research and understand fully why all the medications I took only solved my problems for a few days, and how unhealthy I had been living, and needing laxatives almost every other week, and all my symptoms began to make a lot more sense, I spent a lot of time reading and reading and reading, and when I started to practice everything I had learnt, I became a new person in less than a month, my stomach got flatter, the gas stopped, the belching and acid reflux, the pain too. My skin got better, I got better and more importantly.

It's been about 18 months since I last felt any of these symptoms. My gut health is in perfect condition, and my healing has been permanent.

In this book, I have shared exactly everything I have done that has given me a permanent solution, and no! Not one medication was taken in the course of my recovery. I know it will help you too.

CHAPTER ONE

KNOWING ABOUT YOUR GUT HEALTH

Most people are aware of the importance of the gastrointestinal system to overall health; I wasn't at the time, I wish I did. Either way, it is better to be late than never. You are however, which is a good thing, and that is why you are reading this book.

Your digestive system has been connected in recent years to many other elements of health, including mental stress and long-term conditions like diabetes and cancer. As we now know, the gastrointestinal tract is home to trillions of bacteria that aid in both food digestion and the maintenance of our bodies' general health.

The bacteria and other microorganisms in your stomach and intestines, collectively referred to as your gut (or microbiome) may hold the secret to solving several health problems.

According to studies, gut health can be influenced by specific diets, and habits. This is why it's important to know about your gut health and what you can do to make yours better.

Your gut is the basis for everything. It facilitates food digestion, takes in nutrients, and uses them to power and sustain your body, eliminates pollutants and metabolic waste from your body. Therefore, it will be harder to maintain your health if your immune system and gut are out of balance and your serotonin and hormones aren't functioning properly.

Your body will find it difficult to get rid of those poisons if you have a sick stomach. This can lead to a variety of problems, such as persistent exhaustion, persistent infections, and systemic inflammation. This explains why people have symptoms like gas, diarrhea, constipation, mental fog, joint discomfort, etc. You might not know it, but the brain functions as the second stomach, so when your gut isn't functioning properly, your brain won't either.

The Gut-Brain Connection

There is a serious correlation between the gut and the brain; anxiety can cause stomach issues and vice versa. Have you ever encountered something "gut-wrenching"? Are there circumstances that cause you to "feel like throwing up"? Have you ever had "Butterflies in your belly"? There's a reason we employ these idioms. Emotions can affect the digestive system. Feelings such as anger, worry, grief, and elation, among others, can set off sensations in the gut.

The intestines and stomach are directly impacted by the brain.

For example, just thinking about eating might cause the stomach's contents to flow out before the food does. This relationship is reciprocal. Signals can be used by both a problematic gut and a disturbed brain to communicate with each other.

Therefore, a person's stomach or intestinal issues may cause or result in worry, stress, or sadness. This is because the gastrointestinal (GI) system and the brain are closely related.

This is particularly true when someone has unsettled stomach symptoms without a clear medical reason. It is challenging to attempt gut repair for these functional GI illnesses without taking stress and emotion into account.

The intimate connection between the gut and the brain makes it easy to comprehend why you could experience nausea before a presentation or intestinal pain when under stress. However, this does not imply that functional gastrointestinal disorders are hypothetical or "all in your head."

The causes of pain and other gastrointestinal symptoms include a combination of physical and psychological factors. Both the symptoms and the actual physiology of the gut are influenced by psychosocial factors.

In other words, the GI tract's contractions and movement can be impacted by stress, depression, or other psychological reasons.

Additionally, many patients with functional GI disorders experience pain more intensely than others because their brains are more sensitive to pain signals from the GI tract. Pain that already exists may get worse due to anxiety.

The Digestive System

Food remarkably moves through your body, from the top, which is your mouth, to the bottom, which is your anus. As the beneficial elements in your food are absorbed, you get energy and nutrients. Many organs are involved in your digestive system. Some break down food, while others break down ingested materials like bile.

The network of organs that makes up your digestive system aids in the breakdown and absorption of nutrients from food. It consists of your biliary system and gastrointestinal tract (GI tract). The hollow organs that make up your GI tract are related to one another and extend from your mouth to your anus.

The three organs that make up your biliary system work together to transport bile and digestive enzymes to your GI tract via your bile ducts.

GI tract (gastrointestinal)

Your mouth, esophagus, stomach, small intestine, large intestine, and anus are the organs that comprise your gastrointestinal tract, in the order that they are joined.

The Biliary System

Your pancreas, liver, gallbladder, and bile ducts are all part of your biliary system.

Because of the way it is designed, your digestive system can convert food into the nutrients and energy your body needs to survive.

When it's finished, it neatly compresses your stool, or solid waste, for disposal the next time you have a bowel movement. Water, lipids, proteins, vitamins, and minerals are examples of nutrients.

Nutrients from food and drink are broken down and absorbed by your digestive system so they can be utilized for vital processes including cell growth, repair, and energy production.

This is the way the organs in your digestive system cooperate;

The Mouth

The mouth is where the digestive system begins. In actuality, digestion starts as soon as you bite into something. Your salivary glands get to work once you start eating, you chew your food into smaller, easier-to-digest chunks. Food begins to break down into a form that your body can absorb and use when saliva and food come together.

As you swallow, your tongue pushes the food down your throat and into your esophagus.

The Esophagus

Food passes from your mouth into the esophagus, which is located in your throat near your trachea (windpipe), as you swallow.

The epiglottis is a little flap that covers your windpipe to prevent choking if food lodges in it while swallowing.

Food passes down to your stomach by a process called peristalsis, which is the contraction of the esophageal muscles.

The lower esophageal sphincter, a ring-shaped muscle at the base of the esophagus, must first relax for food to flow through. Subsequently, the sphincter contracts, obstructing the reflux of stomach contents into the esophagus. If it doesn't and the contents flow back into the esophagus, you may have acid reflux or heartburn.

The Stomach

Food is held in the stomach until it is mixed with digestive enzymes, acting as a "container," or hollow organ. The process of converting food into a state that may be ingested is continued by these enzymes. Strong enzymes and acids released by stomach lining cells carry out the breakdown process.

After they have been thoroughly broken down, the contents of the stomach are released into the small intestine.

Pancreatic enzymes and liver bile are used in the meal digestion process. Peristalsis is another way this organ works; it carries food through and combines it with the digestive fluids of the pancreas and liver.

The Intestinal Tract

Comprising three segments—the duodenum, jejunum, and ileum—the small intestine is a muscular tube of 22 feet in length.

The duodenum is the name of the first segment of the small intestine. The continuous breakdown process is primarily its fault. The ileum and jejunum of the lower intestine are principally responsible for absorbing nutrients into the bloodstream.

As they pass through the small intestine, the semi-solid contents finally turn liquid.

The consistency shift is caused by bile, water, mucus, and enzymes. After the nutrients are absorbed, the residual food residue liquid moves from the small intestine into the large intestine (colon).

The Pancreas

Digestive enzymes released by the pancreas break down protein, fats, and carbohydrates in the duodenum. Furthermore, the pancreas produces insulin, which is directly absorbed into the bloodstream. The primary hormone your body needs to digest sugar is insulin.

The Liver

The liver's main function in the digestive system is to process the nutrients that are taken up from the small intestine, while it also does many other things. The breakdown of fat and certain vitamins depends on the bile that the small intestine releases from the liver.

The liver serves as your body's "factory" for chemicals. It uses the basic materials your gut consumes to produce every single chemical your body needs to function.

Furthermore, the liver removes potentially harmful compounds from the body. Numerous drugs that could be detrimental to your health are broken down and secreted by it.

The Gallbladder

To help with fat absorption and digestion, bile from the liver is collected and stored in the gallbladder, which subsequently discharges it into the duodenum in the small intestine.

The Colon

The colon breaks down waste so that emptying your bowels is easy and uncomplicated. The rectum and small intestine are connected by a six-foot-long muscular tube.

The elements that constitute the colon are the cecum, ascending (right), descending (left), transverse (across), and sigmoid (connected to the rectum) colons.

Waste from the digestive process, or stool, is pushed through the colon by the action of peristalsis. It is liquid at first, but it eventually solidifies.

The feces passes through the colon and releases water. A "mass movement" that occurs once or twice a day pushes the contents of the sigmoid (S-shaped) colon into the rectum.

The average time for stool to move through the colon is 36 hours. Bacteria and food scraps make up the majority of the stuff found in feces. In addition to processing food particles and waste products, these "good" bacteria also produce several vitamins and protect the body from pathogens.

The Rectum

Joining the anus and colon lies the rectum, an 8-inch straight chamber. Stools come from the colon, the rectum gathers them, tells you when it has to be evacuated (pooped out) and holds onto them until they are.

When gas or feces enters the rectum, for example, sensors notify the brain. Then the brain decides whether to empty the contents of the rectal cavity or not.

The contents of the rectum are ejected when the rectum contracts and the sphincters relax. If nothing comes out, the sphincter contracts and the rectum expands to make room, easing the pressure for a short while.

The Anus

Anus The appendix represents the final portion of the digestive tract. This 2-inch-long canal is made up of the internal and external anal sphincters, as well as the pelvic floor muscles. The upper anus lining senses the contents of the rectal cavity. It lets you know if what's within is liquid, gas, or solid.

Sphincter muscles surround the anus and are essential for regulating feces. The pelvic floor muscle generates an angle between the rectum and the anus, which prevents stool from coming out when it shouldn't. The internal sphincter is constantly tight unless there is an entering the rectum.

This keeps us continental, preventing us from ejecting gas while we're asleep or in other situations where we wouldn't be aware that we're feces-positive.

The stool is held in place until we use the restroom by our external sphincter, which then relaxes and releases its contents. This helps us control our urge to use the restroom.

Gut health in summary, is the entire wellbeing of these parts, if the well being of one or more is bad, your gut health is bad, a good gut health will indicate that these systems are in perfect health condition, here are some indications that they are not;

Indications That Your Gut health Is Bad

Prolonged Indigestion

Different people define chronic constipation differently. For weeks at a time, infrequent bowel movements are a sign of chronic constipation in certain individuals.

For some, persistent constipation entails straining or experiencing trouble passing stools. For example, a common description of chronic constipation is the sensation that you should be having a bowel movement, but it just won't happen no matter how long you sit.

You may experience little stools, hard or formed stools, or a mix of small, hard, and formed stools on an occasional basis if you have chronic constipation.

For several months, a frequency of fewer than three stools per week is considered chronic constipation. However, this description may not be true because many people who believe they have chronic constipation may underestimate how frequently they go to the bathroom.

Chronic Diarrhea

The usual net absorptive status of water and electrolyte absorption is reversed during diarrhea, leading to secretion.

The elevated water content in the stools (above the normal value of approximately 10 mL/kg/d in infants and young children, or 200 g/d in teenagers and adults) is caused by an imbalance in the physiology of the small and large intestinal processes involved in the absorption of ions, organic substrates, and water.

When three or more loose stools appear suddenly and the episode lasts no more than 14 days, it is referred to as acute diarrhea. When an episode lasts more than 14 days, it is referred to as chronic or persistent diarrhea.

Gas and Bloating

Bloating is a sign of feeling full and confined in your stomach, mainly caused by gas.

Bloating might be confused with other factors that contribute to a bulging abdomen, like the abdominal wall being loose or slack. This is normal, especially for women who are older and have children.

Acid reflux and heartburn

A burning feeling that isn't heartburn but feels like it is in your heart. It is found in the esophagus, the swallowing tube that runs parallel to your heart. The feeling is caused by stomach acid rising to the surface.

Acne and Breakouts

Acne is a skin condition caused by clogged hair follicles filled with dead skin cells and oil. It causes blackheads, whiteheads, or zits. Acne can afflict people of any age, although it most typically affects teenagers. Even while there are effective acne treatments, the condition might occasionally worsen.

Psoriasis and Eczema

When skin cells proliferate more quickly than usual due to immune system stimulation, dead cells accumulate on the skin's surface rather than shedding. This condition is known as psoriasis.

Atopic dermatitis, another name for eczema, is characterized by itching, rashes, swelling, and dryness.

Skin Redness and Rosacea

Rosacea is a chronic inflammatory skin disease that typically affects the nose and cheeks. It creates flushed skin and a rash. Eye issues could also result from it.

The symptoms usually come on and off, and many patients say that particular things, like being in the sun or being under emotional stress, trigger them.

Extended Illness

Chronic fatigue syndrome/myalgic encephalomyelitis (ME/CFS) is a severe, frequently protracted illness that prevents people from engaging in their daily activities. It makes effort, both mental and physical, challenging. Among the symptoms are extreme fatigue, difficulty thinking, and other problems.

Disorientation in the Brain

A common set of symptoms called "brain fog" impairs your ability to focus, recall things, and think clearly. It may make performing daily duties difficult. It is possible to become distracted during a conversation. Though it's usually transient, brain fog can last for a variety of times.

Depression and Anxiety

Mood disorders include depression and anxiety. Depression results in a variety of emotions, including melancholy, hopelessness, and low energy. Anxiety produces uneasiness, concern, or dread. Even if the two prerequisites differ, you can have them both at the same time. Anxiety and melancholy can both be coupled with agitation and restlessness.

Inherent Immune Disorders

Trillions of microorganisms, referred to as the gut microbiota, reside in the gut.

A disruption in the equilibrium of these bacteria can cause dysbiosis, an imbalance associated with autoimmune illnesses, and increase intestinal permeability, which can result in leaky gut syndrome.

Food Intolerances and Allergies

Are dietary sensitivity and allergy the same thing? The phrase "food sensitivity" describes a group of symptoms brought on by an immune system response to certain foods. Generally speaking, these reactions don't get as bad as allergic reactions. Nonetheless, there isn't a precise description of food sensitivity.

Inexplicable Gain in Weight

There is a connection between weight increase and gut bacterial overgrowth. Weight gain may result from an imbalance of gut flora, such as small intestinal bacterial overgrowth (SIBO), which can impair digestion and food absorption.

Challenge in Reducing Body Weight

Based on research, those who are obese may have fewer intestinal flora than moderately weighted persons. Poorer gut health is associated with this.

Researchers have discovered that certain intestinal flora and the ratio of one species of bacteria to another may affect an individual's ability to control their weight.

Hunger and Cravings

Your gut microbiota may go out of balance, which could lead to conflicting messages from your brain about when you're hungry or full. Because the pituitary gland produces hormones that aid in appetite regulation, researchers believe there may be a connection.

PMS and Irregular Menstruation

Gut microorganisms control the amounts of hormone-binding globulins, which in turn control the free levels of the hormone in the bloodstream and are the primary regulator of female sex hormones, particularly estrogen.

Hormone metabolism may be impacted by the gut microbiota. The liver conjugates hormones like estrogen, progesterone, and testosterone, and the gut flora is crucial to the excretion process. These hormone levels may be impacted by unbalanced microbiomes, which could result in irregular menstruation or hormonal imbalances.

Failing Thyroid

Individuals with thyroid conditions, such as Graves' disease and Hashimoto's thyroiditis (more on these below), frequently have gut dysbiosis. Inflammation and "leaky gut" can be caused by poor thyroid function, which in turn can be impacted by poor gut health.

CHAPTER TWO

HOW TO REPAIR YOUR GUT HEALTH

You've undoubtedly read a ton of articles, books and watched videos about improving your gut health; many herbs and supplements have been suggested, and you may even have tried a few. However, as everything ultimately comes down to what you consume in your mouth, these four easy ways to improve the health of your gut won't fail.

Simple Steps to Repair Your Gut Permanently:

1. Elimination
2. Repair
3. Re-introduce
4. Maintenance

The Elimination Stage

When I was plagued with consistent bloating and constipation that came with a lot of abdominal pain, I just knew I had to find a permanent solution to my problems, instead of popping pills after pills, laxatives and herbal teas after eating a tiny morsel of food. I knew I couldn't continue to live that way, the constant flatulence too made it hard for me to socialize, not to mention the bad stench from belching I frequently had. It was this struggle that made me take out 6 months to fully research about what was causing my symptoms and how I could live without those discomfort without medication orthodox or unorthodox, as these medications were temporal fixes. It didn't take long before I discovered first that I had to clear out my gut, and follow it up with other helpful steps. These steps made me free in 28 days.

Elimination is the first step, here you get rid of the causes and triggers.

Understanding the underlying causes of poor gut health is necessary before taking effective action to eradicate the causes. Eating foods that negatively impact your gut microbiota can produce imbalances, inflammation, and a higher risk of digestive problems including irritable bowel syndrome (IBS). This is only one of many core causes.

The top ten foods that are detrimental to gut health include but not limited to;

1. Processed meals

The gut microbiome can be harmed by processed foods since they are heavy in harmful fats, preservatives, and additives.

2. Refined sugar

Refined sugar can cause inflammation and digestive problems by upsetting the balance of microorganisms in your stomach.

3. Gluten

Gluten is a protein that can lead to intestinal inflammation in those who have non-celiac gluten sensitivity or celiac disease. It is found in wheat, barley, and rye.

4. Products made from dairy

Dairy products can trigger digestive problems including gas, bloating, and diarrhea in a lot of people.

5. Fried foods

Fried meals contain a lot of bad fats, which can damage your gut flora and cause inflammation.

6. Flesh from red meat

Eating red meat regularly raises the risk of colon cancer and can cause inflammation.

7. Synthetic sugar substitutes

Artificial sweeteners have the potential to upset your gut's bacterial balance and aggravate digestive problems.

8. Tobacco

Too much Tobacco can damage your gut microbiota, which can cause immune system decline and digestive problems.

9. Coffee

While a reasonable amount of caffeine is usually harmless, too much of it can lead to stomach problems including acid reflux and heartburn.

10. Corn syrup with high fructose

High-fructose corn syrup is a highly processed sugar that can cause inflammation and upset your gut's bacterial balance.

Additionally, routines, and habits, such as these, can also affect your gut health:

- You Take Substances That Impair Your Digestive System

Certain medications may cause serious harm to your gut microbiota. One medication that is regularly given is an antibiotic. Prescription antibiotics are used to remove pathogenic or harmful bacteria from your body so that you can recover from illness.

But keep in mind that antibiotics often destroy beneficial bacteria in addition to pathogenic or "bad" germs!

Probiotics are advised as a result of following an antibiotic course.

It's also critical to note that a lot of animal products include antibiotics.

You unintentionally introduce them to your microbiome and compromise the health of your gut when you consume any animal products because they are fed to animals and added to their feed to prevent infection.

Other drugs that may cause an imbalance in your stomach are:

Proton pump inhibitors (PPIs), which are used to treat acid reflux, ulcers, and dyspepsia, laxatives, and Oral contraceptives also affect the intestinal flora of women

- You're Not Sleeping Enough

Everybody has experienced sleepless evenings that left them feeling drowsy and irritable the following day. I think any mother out there is familiar with this emotion! Your general health depends greatly on getting enough sleep and having a restful night's sleep. It's also crucial for the health of your digestive system.

When you don't get enough sleep, your stomach suffers problems with intestinal permeability and leaky gut syndrome. Your stress levels may rise if you don't get enough sleep. Gut permeability problems such as leaky gut syndrome can be brought on by elevated stress.

Your body's normal melatonin production can be harmed and cortisol, the stress hormone, can rise as a result of little sleep. The hormone that is often associated with sleep, melatonin, also controls the motility of your gastrointestinal tract. In other words, it facilitates the smooth passage of food through your digestive system. You can be more prone to heartburn or acid reflux when you're trying to go to sleep if this is off.

- Excessive smoking habits

There are thousands of compounds in tobacco smoke, and 70 of those can cause cancer.

Smoking damages almost all of the body's organs and increases the chance of lung cancer, heart disease, and stroke.

One of the most significant environmental risk factors for inflammatory bowel disease, which is defined by persistent inflammation of the digestive tract, is cigarette smoking.

Moreover, compared to non-smokers, smokers have a double higher risk of developing Crohn's disease, a prevalent form of inflammatory bowel illness.

One study found that quitting smoking enhanced the diversity of gut flora, a sign of a healthy stomach.

- Eating Late

Eating too soon before bed can cause stagnation and poor digestion.

This is a serious issue, particularly if you habitually stay up late.

When you eat right before bed, your body uses up vital energy digesting the meal instead of attempting to fall asleep!

- Excessive Alcohol Consumption

When ingested in excess, alcohol can have negative physical and psychological effects in addition to being highly poisonous and addictive.

Chronic alcohol usage can lead to major issues with gut health, such as dysbiosis.

In one study, 10 healthy people who drank little to no alcohol were compared to 41 alcoholics to see what kind of gut flora they had. Of the people who were alcoholics, 27% had dysbiosis, while none of the healthy people had it.

Three different types of alcohol were examined in terms of their effects on gut health in another study.

Each person drank 9.2 ounces (272 ml) of red wine, the same volume of red wine that has been de-alcoholized, or 3.4 ounces (100 ml) of gin every day for 20 days.

Red wine boosted the abundance of bacteria known to support gut health and lowered the number of hazardous gut bacteria like Clostridium, while gin decreased the number of good gut bacteria.

Its polyphenol concentration appears to be the reason why moderate red wine drinking is good for gut flora.

Plant chemicals called polyphenols are broken down by intestinal bacteria after evading digestion. Additionally, they might lower blood pressure and raise cholesterol.

- Infrequent Exercise

Simply put, physical activity is any bodily action that results in energy burn.

Physical activities include swimming, cycling, gardening, and walking.

There are several health advantages to physical activity, such as decreased stress levels, weight loss, and a lesser chance of chronic illness.

Furthermore, new research indicates that exercise may change gut flora to improve gut health.

Greater amounts of butyrate-producing bacteria and butyrate, a short-chain fatty acid vital to general health, have been linked to higher fitness levels.

Professional rugby players, when compared to control groups matched for body size, age, and gender, had twice as many different bacterial families and more diverse gut flora, according to one study.

Athletes also exhibited larger concentrations of Akkermansia, a bacterium that has been linked to metabolic health and the avoidance of obesity.

In one study, the gut flora of 19 physically active women and 21 inactive women were compared.

Bifidobacterium and Akkermansia, two bacteria that promote health, were more prevalent in active women, indicating that frequent physical activity, even at low-to-moderate intensities, can be advantageous.

In conclusion, regular exercise encourages the development of Bifidobacterium and Akkermansia, two types of good gut bacteria. Those who are not active do not experience these benefits.

- Overwhelming Stress

It takes more than just a balanced diet, regular exercise, and enough sleep to be healthy.

Excessive levels of stress can also be detrimental to one's health. Stress can change the gut's flora, decrease blood flow, and enhance sensitivity.

Research on mice has demonstrated that a variety of stressors, including heat stress, crowding, and isolation, can change gut profiles and limit the diversity of gut flora.

Stress exposure also has an impact on the populations of bacteria, leading to a decrease in Lactobacillus populations and an increase in potentially dangerous bacteria like Clostridium.

In a human investigation, the impact of stress on the makeup of 23 college students' gut microbes was examined.

As earlier stated, in order to effectively carry out the elimination phase of repairing your gut health, you have to first identify what to eliminate.

Now, when it comes to food and gut health, you are likely eating so many things at a time. This would make it a little more difficult to pinpoint which foods in particular are causing you more harm than good, you may or may not be allergic to dairy products, and the same goes for gluten.

But with the list above, you can narrow down and eliminate them in the first 10 days of your recovery process.

You will gradually remove each of these eating patterns and habits, and foods that support poor gut health during the elimination phase.

During the elimination stage, you would cut out dairy and gluten even if you are not sure you respond negatively to them. You should be able to do this in 10 days. This will give your digestive system a chance to reset so you may go on to the healing stage. In the maintenance stage, you can progressively reintroduce dairy and gluten one at a time to see how your body responds to them before determining whether to exclude them entirely from your diet or not.

The Repair Stage

The repair stage, actually started from the elimination stage, I make it bold to say that the body is the most complex, most sophisticated machine there is, and it self repairs it self, and the majority of the damage that happens in our bodies, happen due to doing too much of the wrong things to it, or not doing enough of the right things, in your gut repair journey, the repair will start the day you start to eliminate the triggers of bad gut health.

However, to make repair and healing faster, you will have to introduce foods and habits that are good for your gut health.

So, in the repair stage, you'll be focused on;

    A. Gut healing foods
    B. Lifestyle Changes

Gut Health Healing Foods

Aside from a few better behaviors, you will give specific "gut healing foods," as I like to call them, priority during the healing period.

I would divide these foods that cure the gut into 3 categories:

1. Probiotics rich meals
2. Fiber rich meals/Vegetables and fruits
3. Whole foods
4. Hydration - Water

Probiotics Rich Meals

Numerous bacteria are beneficial to human health, despite the common misconception that they are dangerous pathogens that contaminate food or cause illness. In addition to breaking down and absorbing food, the human gut is home to trillions of bacteria and other microbes that are vital to our continued health.

Probiotics are "good" microbes that can be found in supplements or dietary items. They can enhance the equilibrium of intestinal flora, which is beneficial to our health. They come in a variety of formats, including sachets, tablets, yogurts, and capsules.

Probiotics can assist your body in various ways to ensure optimal performance by balancing the intestinal flora.

When you eat them, they drive out potentially dangerous bacteria from your stomach by competing with them for nutrients and space. Additionally, probiotics strengthen your immune system's ability to combat infections.

For instance, research has indicated that they may shorten the duration of colds and enhance your body's reaction to some vaccinations.

To maintain a healthy gut lining, probiotics can also aid in the production of acid molecules and aid in the digestion of fiber.

Many studies have been conducted to determine the benefits of probiotic use for both healthy individuals and those with particular conditions. These are a few situations where probiotics may be helpful, although the scientific evidence supporting their use is continually expanding.

Probiotics have a lot of potential health benefits when added to the diet. One of the best foods to get probiotics in is yogurt. Probiotics can also be found in kimchi, pickles, kombucha, miso, sauerkraut, and other foods. Recall that certain probiotic foods may contain dairy.

During your repair stage, you should only use probiotics that are not dairy foods. Afterward, you can progressively reintroduce the probiotics that are dairy foods during the reintroduction stage and observe how your body responds.

Fiber Rich Meals

Dietary fiber softens and makes your feces heavier and bigger. Because a thick stool is easier to pass, constipation is less likely to occur.

Fiber can help stabilize loose, watery stools because it absorbs water and gives the stool bulk. Preserves intestinal health.

Fiber: Soluble vs. Insoluble
Because soluble fibers of all kinds slow down digestion, the body takes longer to absorb sugar, or glucose, from the food you eat. Preventing abrupt increases in blood sugar levels is crucial for the effective management of diabetes.

Additionally, fatty acids and soluble fibers bond, removing them from the body and assisting in the reduction of LDL (bad) cholesterol. These kinds of fiber-rich foods include apples, blueberries, almonds, beans, and oatmeal.

Insoluble fibers aid in the digestion and passage of waste via your intestines. This keeps you regular by preventing constipation. Fruit skins and seeds contain insoluble fiber, so always consume the peels. In addition, whole wheat bread, brown rice, and leafy greens like kale contain it.

Consuming a diverse range of veggies is beneficial to your general well-being. In particular, vegetables such as bean sprouts, lettuce, peas, mushrooms, and baby spinach can help improve the health of your gut. These veggies are excellent for your digestive system because they are high in fiber, water, or plant chemicals called polyphenols. There are times when all three are combined.

Certain veggies are more strongly linked to "good" gut flora than others, according to our findings.

The top ten veggies for intestinal health are as follows:

Fungi

Cucumber

Little watercress with spinach leeks

Sprouting beans

Lettuce

Green beans

Asparagus and cauliflower

1. fungi

Spores are produced by mushrooms, which is the portion of the fungus that facilitates its reproduction. Mushrooms come in a variety of tasty varieties that are also very beneficial to intestinal health.

Mushrooms are on this list because they offer many of the same health advantages as vegetables, while not being considered vegetables per se.

A 2017 research found that a variety of chemicals found in mushrooms function as prebiotics for your gut microbiota. Prebiotics are nutrients that support the growth of your "good" bacteria. They frequently take the shape of fiber.

The bacteria in our stomachs break down fiber to create substances known as short-chain fatty acids. These give your gut's lining cells energy. They also strengthen the "good" bacteria that already reside in your stomach and mend the barrier. The uses for mushrooms are endless. You can bake, fry, or BBQ them, based on your preferred texture. They complement nearly any herb or spice and provide sauces and soups with a rich, earthy umami flavor.

2. Peeled cucumbers

Technically speaking, cucumbers are a kind of berry. Nonetheless, they are on this list since most people consider them to be vegetables. The bacteria in your stomach can consume a variety of plant chemicals found in cucumbers. Among these substances are polyphenols, a class of molecules that may aid in promoting the development of "good" gut flora.

A 2022 review suggests that these plant components may also have antioxidant properties and prevent the growth of "bad" microorganisms.

Moreover, water makes up more than 96% of a cucumber. Additionally, drinking enough water helps keep your stools smooth and stave against constipation. Cucumbers pair well with soups and dips in addition to traditional salads.

3. Baby spinach

Farmers harvest baby spinach, a leafy green, earlier off the vine than mature spinach.

It's loaded with iron, calcium, and other minerals, as well as vitamins A, C, and K, and polyphenols.

Baby spinach is more than just a base for salads; it can also be used as a base for stir-fries, soups, and sauces. It can even be layered into lasagnas. You can usually get a lot of spinach for your money if you choose frozen. Additionally, producers freeze veggies soon after they are harvested, preserving a wealth of nutrients that might otherwise be lost over time.

4. The watercress
This herbaceous, spicy green thrives in organic mineral water. It offers vital elements including iron and phosphorus along with vitamins A, B1, B2, C, and E.
According to a 2021 study, the plant is also beneficial for digestive health because it includes a variety of polyphenols known as flavonoids.

With little preparation needed, watercress may infuse flavor into soups, sandwiches, and sauces. It can also give pesto and dips a richer flavor.

5. Onions

Though they are a little sweeter, leeks belong to the same family as onions. They supply inulin, a fiber that is a naturally occurring prebiotic. According to a 2023 review, inulin may also help you absorb more nutrients from your diet and ease constipation.

Leeks are a staple in soups and stews, and the entire vegetable can be used in cooking. You can roast or sauté them, but they're also good eaten raw.

6. Sprouting beans

The young, edible sprouts of the mung bean are called bean sprouts. They can be found in Thai, Korean, Chinese, and Indian cuisines.

Just one 115-gram cup of cooked bean sprouts contains 3.8 g of fiber, making these sprouts an excellent source of fiber. Regardless of age or gender, that is more than 10% of the daily fiber intake that is advised.

Specifically, sprouting beans are an excellent source of insoluble fiber. Not soluble in water, this variety facilitates the passage of food through the digestive system and wards off constipation. Additionally, bean sprouts include polyphenols that support the "good" flora in your stomach. Simply wash some sprouts and add them to a curry or stir-fry for added crunch and digestive health advantages.

7. Romaine

Carotenoids and polyphenols are beneficial components of lettuce. Varieties differ in terms of nutrient content, texture, and color. Additionally, lettuce contains a lot of water—roughly 94–95%—and hydration is essential for healthy digestion. Aside from salads, lettuce works well in soups and burritos.

Alternatively, you can make wraps or burgers with lettuce leaves in place of the bread.

8. Peas in the green

When peas reach maturity, they resemble beans more than vegetables. However, starchy veggies can include the green peas in your freezer. They produce pods when they ripen. Certain types, like snow peas, are edible in their pods; however, other varieties, like garden peas, which are sold in bags without pods, are not. One cup of green peas provides 8.6 g of fiber, making them an excellent source of fiber.

This fiber, about 6 g of it, is insoluble, which facilitates food passage through the digestive tract and lowers the chance of constipation. There is still 2.6 g that is soluble.

In your stomach, soluble fiber turns into a gel-like material when it dissolves in water. It thickens and softens feces, slows down digestion, and traps cholesterol in the gut to prevent it from entering the bloodstream.

To make a side dish that goes well with any protein or starch, just sauté green peas in butter over medium heat with a dash of salt.

9. Zucchini

The skin, meat, and seeds of the zucchini plant, also called a courgette, resemble cucumbers and are edible. This variety of summer squash contains some soluble and insoluble fiber and is 94% water. Therefore, zucchini provides both types of gut-supporting fiber and aids in keeping us hydrated. Add sautéed, roasted, or fried zucchini to stir-fries, salads, and sauces. You can also make zucchini noodles as a high-fiber, low-carb alternative to pasta.

10. Lettuce

In reality, the "head" of cauliflower that you eat is a half-formed flower. The most popular kind of cauliflower is white, but you may also try orange, purple, and green kinds. 92-14% of fresh cauliflower is water. Its fiber content is also very high—2.14 g of fiber per cup (107 g). The key benefit of cauliflower is its adaptability.

Its subtle flavor makes it suitable for frying, baking, or steaming. Cauliflower is great in salads, soups, and curries, but it can also be used as a low-carb base for pizza. It can also be used to "rice" or to make vegan chicken wings.

Consuming an adequate amount of fiber can help you maintain weight control, regulate your bowel motions, and reduce your chance of contracting specific illnesses.

When attempting to eat healthfully, it's simple to become engrossed in tracking calories and grams of added sugars, fats, proteins, and carbohydrates. However, dietary fiber is one nutrient that is all too frequently overlooked.

The health benefits of consuming fiber have long been recognized by scientists. You need big hospitals if you pass little stools. Years later, many of us are still neglecting to consume enough fiber.

Regretfully, most of us barely consume roughly half of the recommended daily amount of fiber and even less of the incredibly healthy fructans.

However, there is good news: research published in the journal Nature found that increasing your fiber consumption can quickly improve your gut flora—sometimes in as little as five days.

Just keep in mind to go slowly. By gradually increasing your fiber intake, you can prevent bloating and gas.

Whole foods

In a nutshell, whole foods are those that have undergone either little or no processing. Whole grains, legumes, and fresh fruits and vegetables are a few examples. Consider items whose labels don't need to disclose a million different, difficult-to-pronounce substances.

This indicates that rather than being an afterthought, plants—vegetables, fruits, whole grains, legumes, beans, seeds, and nuts—are the main contents of your diet.

It only requires that you consume proportionately more vegetables; it doesn't require you to be vegan or even vegetarian.

When you shop for food, choose items that are as close to or in their natural state as possible. Among the things to avoid are processed oils, flour, and added sugars. Select pressed coconut or extra virgin olive oils over processed ones whenever you can.

Inarguably, whole foods provide more nutrition, the ideal base for optimum health is a diet rich in nutrients, not supplements. As nature intended, entire foods provide all the nutrients we require without the use of additives. We're covering all the bases whcn wc consume a range of fruits, vegetables, whole grains, and protein-rich foods regularly. Furthermore, even these so-called "protein foods" should mostly consist of plant-based foods; tempeh and tofu are excellent meat alternatives and are considered whole foods.

If you base your diet mostly on plant-based foods, you will inevitably ingest:

The majority of vitamins and minerals, if not all of them, are essential for optimal bodily function; the most important one to be aware of is vitamin B12, Dietary fiber, which keeps your digestive system functioning properly, minimum amounts of trans and saturated fats, unsaturated fats, and zero cholesterol, an abundance of protein, amongst many other essential nutrients.

The substances that function as a plant's immune system are called phytonutrients. Among them are antioxidants, which also aid in the battle against human disease.

If you find it hard to eat more whole foods, and rather convenient to eat junk and processed foods, here is how to consume more complete meals.

Firstly, see eating whole foods more as a way of life, instead of a chore. Try to keep dry and frozen goods on hand.

It's not always necessary to buy whole items fresh; dry lentils and frozen vegetables also function well.

Make a plan beforehand, preparing ahead is one of the simplest methods to start including more whole foods in your weekly routine, even though it does require some time and work.

We typically make less conscious (and frequently unhealthy) decisions while we're rushing or on the go. Being organized aids with maintaining attention.

Begin with a single daily meal, if organizing your entire week seems too restrictive or overwhelming, consider just organizing one wholesome whole-food meal every day. This is a terrific place to start.

Displace animal-based products, as you actively begin to move your focus away from animal products, you will naturally increase the proportion of plants you eat, whether your goal is to eat all plants or just more of them. Half of your plate should consist of fruits and/or vegetables, 25% should be whole grains, and 25% should be protein-rich foods, and to your heart's content, season away.

Furthermore, whole foods do not have to be boring. In general, entire foods are used to make spices, herbs, and seasonings; however, condiments like mustard, salsa, nutritional yeast, soy sauce, vinegar, and lemon juice are also recommended.

4. Hydration - Water.

Additionally, a 2022 study discovered that a certain type of bacteria linked to gastrointestinal diseases was less common in those who drank more water. Drinking adequate water has benefits for general health and can help prevent constipation. It may also be a simple way to maintain gut health.

Lifestyle Changes

You have probably read a lot about how the gut health depends on what you eat, while this is not far from the truth, remember we talked about the gut-mind connection, it is not only food that affects your gut health, and the sole priority of this book is to help you repair your gut permanently, which is why we will also tackled other factors that affect gut health, like one's habits and lifestyle.

In this section however, I will be sharing effective techniques to help you manage these habits and lifestyle, these techniques include;

Techniques for Reducing Stress

Whatever the source of stress, it's critical to take into account how stress affects your overall health and well-being. After all, excessive stress can have detrimental effects on your body, both mentally and physically, including disrupting your digestion and gut.

The impact that stress has on your digestive system varies depending on how long it lasts:

Stress that lasts only a short while can make you less hungry and slow down your digestion.

Prolonged stress can lead to gastrointestinal (GI) problems such as upset stomach, constipation, diarrhea, or indigestion.

Extended durations of chronic stress have been linked to more significant conditions such as GI problems and irritable bowel syndrome.

Consistent stress reduction is one of the secrets to improved digestion. Reducing stress allows your body to concentrate on absorbing the nutrients you require, which can reduce inflammation in the gut, improve GI distress, and keep you nourished.

These four suggestions will help you heal your gut if you notice that your stress levels are interfering with your digestion.

Do yoga.

Make sure you engage in regular physical activity, such as walking and jogging, to improve and support your digestion.

In addition to focusing on alignment and posture, exercises like Hatha or Iyengar, yoga may help reduce gastrointestinal symptoms and enhance stress results.

3 Yoga Asanas to Encourage Indigestion;

1. Try practicing mindful meditation.

According to scientific studies, practicing mindful meditation, which entails increasing your awareness of your everyday life, may also be beneficial.

2. Deep breathing exercises

Deep breathing exercises and meditation may reduce inflammation, which is the body's indicator of stress. Consequently, this could alleviate an overworked digestive system.

3. Sitting up straight

Try sitting up straight away from distractions before your next meal, and do two or four rounds of deep breathing. taking four breaths, holding each for four counts, and then letting go for four counts.

To assist your body relax and prepare for digestion, do this every time you sit down to eat (i.e. rest and digest mode).

Give up Smoking

When your stress level is rising and you find yourself reaching for a cigarette, it's time to reconsider this coping mechanism.

Cigarette smoking is most widely linked to heart disease and respiratory disorders, but studies also indicate that unhealthy habits might have an impact on your digestive system.

Smoking raises the chance of stomach ulcers, gastrointestinal disorders, and cancers associated with them.

Many people attempt to stop smoking on their own, but with the correct support, quitting smoking is considerably simpler. There are plenty of resources available to support you as you embark on your quitting journey. You may wish to think about the side effects and the price of smoking. If you've tried to quit in the past, consider the strategies that will work for you and any changes you might want to make.

The secret is to persevere and try several combinations until you discover the one that suits you best.

Some tips for quitting

Here are some pointers to get you there.

- Don't forget to put your chosen quit date in your calendar when you've chosen it.
- List out your reasons for quitting
- Inform others that you're giving up.
- Recall what worked if you've attempted to stop previously.
- Make use of cessation tools.
- When you are tempted to smoke, have a strategy.
- List the things that make you want to smoke and ways to avoid them.
- Stay occupied to ward off cravings.
- Get moving to stifle the impulse.

Rest Effectively

An increasing number of people these days seem to have forgotten how to fully unwind. Neither workers nor students have enough time for rest periods or enough sleep.

Many people experience fatigue even after taking a holiday or vacation. Overworking has progressively taken the place of a more balanced lifestyle that includes regular downtime.

For this reason, in this book:
You'll discover solutions to deal with tiredness. I have compiled a wealth of practical advice on how to relax well. You won't experience low motivation or productivity after implementing our resting habits suggestions into your everyday routine.

Give up on social media.
When they have a moment to spare, a lot of people launch their social network applications automatically. This is not a good method to unwind. We'll go over the reasons it's best to avoid staring at your phone while taking a break. So what damage might come from browsing social media while taking a break from work or studying?

Your mind never shuts off. Artificial stimulation is found in movies, video games, television, and social media. Your brain is not at rest when you perform these tasks. Even though the material is interesting, it is being inundated and becoming increasingly weary. Your brain needs downtime because it is a muscle as well. Give it some time to relax so that when you need it to operate, it will do so quite well.

You become anxious. Because social media is so widely used and available, we usually feel as though we must constantly check our newsfeeds. The stress hormone cortisol may be released into our bodies more frequently as a result of this sense of duty. Depression or even memory loss may result from elevated cortisol levels. In general, you feel less anxious the more you avoid social media.

You stay up late using social media. Before turning in for the night, scrolling through phones is a frequent practice. You may not even realize how fast an hour or two goes by.

Try reading a book or practicing meditation before turning in instead of browsing social media.

You grow weary of it. Excessive time spent on social media might be tiresome or frustrating. Scrolling through your newsfeed without purpose can quickly get monotonous. You could try reading a book, doing a crossword puzzle, or doing other hobbies that comfortably stimulate your brain.

Concentrating on oneself gets challenging. We'll go into more detail on why it's important to take time for yourself during a study or work break in the sections that follow. Social media platforms let you notice other people. Developing and comprehending your thoughts can be challenging when you read other people's comments and look at their photographs. You'll learn more about yourself if you put others out of your mind.

Having said that, I am not suggesting that you give up on social media completely; that is a subject for a different conversation. We do, however, advise you to restrict the amount of time you spend online during a break from work or school. If you want to keep your drive and productivity levels up, you must give your brain a break.

Practice meditation
When someone mentions meditation, have you ever seen them roll their eyes? They frequently underestimate its true strength for unknown reasons. The best method to unwind and clear your mind of stress and pointless information is to practice meditation. This section will explain how.

In general, wherever you are (at work or home), there are a lot of different techniques to meditate. The following components comprise the majority of the method.

Focus

Focus your concentration during your meditation. It will support you in avoiding distractions and maintaining an uncluttered, worry-free mind.

Serene location

When it comes to meditation, setting is important. If you're just starting, pick a calm, cozy area. You can practice meditation anywhere—in a traffic jam, in a queue at the store, etc.—once you learn it.

Inhaling deeply

Take in enough oxygen and calm down your breathing as you meditate. Your muscles will become more relaxed, and your mind will be revitalized.

A suitable stance

Before you begin your meditation, make sure you are in the correct position. You should be at ease whether you are sitting, standing, or lying down. You won't be able to focus otherwise.

Positivity in outlook

Take in some good energy and let your thoughts flow. After you meditate, you'll realize how much more at ease you feel.

Set Up Your Office

You have likely done some work or studied from home throughout the pandemic. You must also have learned that a well-organized workspace should be kept apart from other zones. You'll see why it's essential for your sleep and rest here.

Motives for devoting time to creating your ideal workspace:

Your quality of sleep will improve. Generally, you think of your bed when you think of comfort and sleep. One is more prone to eventually have insomnia or fall asleep when working or studying in bed. A better night's sleep is also achieved by keeping computers and other work- or school-related materials away from the bed.

You must relocate and alter your surroundings to relax after studying or working. This isn't always feasible, though, particularly during a pandemic. It's crucial to pay close attention to the workplace during these stressful times.

Give Up Wearing Yourself Out
You won't get enough sleep if you work too much. You run a higher risk of burnout and other mental and health problems when you overextend yourself.

Working excessive hours can result in uninspired work and subpar results. It is therefore preferable to quit when it is appropriate. You should put off doing your responsibilities till the next day if you feel like you're almost at your breaking point. It's preferable to leave things partially completed since you'll continue to think about them subconsciously and come up with better solutions.

How can you recognize when you're worn out? How do you decide when to put in your workday and take a break? Look for these indicators, and ideally stop working before they show up:

Physical Indications
Signs of Emotion
Action Marks
Pain, sleeplessness
Absence of drive or output
Subpar work performance
Upset stomach, altered appetite, and fluctuations in weight
Depression
unable to fulfill obligations, whether personal or professional
Persistent exhaustion and rising sickness
Feelings of hopelessness and apathy
Loneliness and lack of social contact

Schedule Your Vacations

We always plan our work, workouts, and get-togethers with friends and coworkers. However, we frequently neglect to schedule breaks. And it is the biggest error we made! It is also advisable to plan for rest. I'll explain why in this section.

In your calendar, you should identify the appropriate time for: Ten to fifteen minutes every two hours; A minimum of one hour for the midday meal. And never pass them by.

Exercise Frequently

I can now go on to more useful guidance. More specifically, what to do with your free time when social media and the Internet aren't available. Exercise is the first piece of advice I have for you. Feel-good molecules are activated when you exercise. While your body may feel exhausted, your mind will begin to unwind. That is how the human body works.

Additionally, doing sports relieves stress. Serotonin, the pleasure hormone, is released by our brain during exercise and lowers cortisol levels, which helps treat depression.

I advise you to visit the gym during your lunch break for the reasons mentioned above.

However, given the times, it might not be feasible. So, the following advice can help you work out at home.

Plan out your exercise. We learn from time management that weekly activity planning is crucial. You will be more driven to complete your tasks when you have allocated a definite time. Take a look at some sample training plans if you're unsure about how to organize your own.

Find a suitable place to work out. Pick a space in your home that is at least the size of a yoga mat for your workout. Don't pick a room for your consideration that you also use for eating or sleeping. In this manner, you will resist the need to pause and grab a quick snack or binge-watch some Netflix.

Modify your objectives. You shouldn't begin heavy lifting as soon as you start exercising. Always pay attention to your body and start cautiously. Never forget to take it easy on yourself if you want to enjoy your downtime.

Choose ten different workouts. Select ten primary workouts that range in intensity. You could wish to combine some easier exercises like jumping jacks. Additionally, consider including some stretching, strength training, and core exercises.

Assign a timer. Exercise regimens for beginners may require less time than for seasoned practitioners.

Recall not to exert too much pressure. Now is the time to move comfortably and give your mind a break. So begin your warm-up by turning on your favorite tune. And relish your exercise! Our essay collection has many articles on the subject of exercise, so you may discover additional information there.

Take a stroll

Do you dislike working out at a high intensity when you're taking a break? I have a suggestion for you instead: take a stroll! You can revitalize your entire body and mind with this exercise. We'll explain why it's worthwhile, so don't worry.

You'll become more effective. People often become distracted and less motivated to complete tasks by midday. It will therefore be advantageous to go for a quick stroll following lunch. You'll experience a mental and physical renewal as well as a boost in productivity.

Walking lifts your spirits. Did you know that when you engage in physical activity, your body releases endorphins? That's why taking a walk improves your mood. Imagine feeling better and better with each step.

It facilitates restful sleep. Lack of sleep is arguably the most prevalent issue among individuals with busy schedules. Taking a stroll during the day or right before bed is an easy way to tackle this issue. Your sleep will become significantly better.

It's simple and soothing. This is not an activity that requires extra effort on your part. All you have to do is get out of bed and walk outside. As easy as that! Nonetheless, you'll find that your body becomes more in harmony and that your mind is revitalized.

You'll become more fit. Living a sedentary lifestyle can have a lot of negative effects on your health. Remember that mobility is the essence of life! Take a quick stroll as part of your everyday regimen. It will help you maintain your physical fitness and—more significantly—avoid chronic illnesses like diabetes, hypertension, etc.

To maximize the advantages of spending time outside, you can do some or all of these;

- Visit a park.
- Enjoy some light music or the sounds of nature.
- Avoid doing active thinking.
- Engage in mindfulness.

What kind of exercise is necessary to have a healthier digestive system? Engage in any kind of aerobic activity that suits your fitness level and timetable.

People think they have to join a class when they hear the word aerobic, but that's not the case. You can get in an aerobic workout by raking leaves, vacuuming the living room, cutting the grass, or dancing to your favorite music.

How can you know if the level of intensity you're working out at is appropriate? Watch out for these warning signs:

- Your heart rate is higher than usual. You
- speak, but you can't sing.
- You're starting to sweat.

Your target should be 30 minutes of exercise five days a week. If you don't succeed in reaching your goal, nevertheless, don't give up. It is better to engage in any activity than none at all.

Many people get frustrated when they miss a few days of exercise. But regardless of how that looks, the important thing is to move as much as you can.

Take it slow at first.

If you're new to exercising, be cautious not to overdo it and get hurt.

Don't do too much, too soon—this can strain muscles or hurt yourself. You are at the proper intensity as long as your heart rate is elevated.

Don't push yourself past your comfort zone or you risk getting yourself back.

When dealing with cardiac issues, exercise caution. See your doctor before starting any kind of exercise if you have a heart or lung issue.

While raising your heart rate is generally a good thing, it might not be safe with certain heart conditions. You can choose the right kind of exercise by consulting with your healthcare provider.

Your body will appreciate you for it, stomach included, no matter how you decide to move.

Exercise is one of the most powerful ways to improve your overall health, including your gut health. Almost anyone can do it, and it doesn't have to cost anything, to feel better.

The Re-introduction Stage

I am of the opinion that, except that something is poisonous and concerns you harm, there's no reason to not enjoy the foods that you love.

Not all foods with bad PR are bad, they are just consumed excessively, not balanced out or not consumed enough.

So, in the re-introduction stage, after your symptoms have completely ceased and you are starting to feel like yourself again, You should start to reintroduce dairy products little by little and carefully observe how your body reacts to them. This should be done around the last 7 days of your gut repair journey.

In my case, as someone who loved eggs, bread, milk and yogurt and was hitting the gym, and needed affordable and rich sources of protein, I had to try again to see if I really was allergic to dairy products.

So, I would include one dairy product every 2 days and observe.

If your symptoms return, you can stop them completely and look for their plant replacements.

You should also do this for gluten products and finally stick to a healthier diet that is suitable for your health.

The Maintenance Stage

Now that your health is getting better, you have identified the triggers, and sieved out the meals that were causing you harm, to keep your results permanent would depend on how you live your life moving forward.

Your diet, your habits and lifestyle. If you relapse and go back to the old foods you used to eat, and the habits you used to keep, your gut will suffer once more.

I will be sharing some tips to help you stay consistent.

1. Start with modest dietary adjustments.

It's normal to be ecstatic about your newfound health and desire to drastically change your diet. However, making too many changes too quickly increases the risk of burnout and completely quitting your healthy routines.

Advice: To gradually improve your nutrition, set modest goals for each week. For instance, try having a plate of vegetables with dinner instead of white toast for breakfast.

2. Consume meals that are balanced and filling.

When weight loss is the aim, it can be tempting to micromanage portions or avoid carbohydrates. But to feel in control of your eating and feel fuller for longer, it's critical to consume enough food—and enough of the correct kinds of food.

Advice: Make sure that the majority of your meals contain protein, carbs, and fats. It's preferable if you can increase your intake of fiber by eating more fruits, veggies, and whole grains!

3. Eat at regular intervals during the day.

Refusing meals and snacks seems like a simple approach to reducing caloric intake. However, the likelihood is that it will make you feel extremely agitated and compulsive over food.

Advice: Give up missing meals and snacks. Try to find an eating schedule that fits in with your schedule and try to eat every three to four hours.

4. Give up taking cheat days.

It's wonderful to find a healthy balance, but cheat days aren't the way to get there. Cheat days encourage overeating, keep you trapped in the all-or-nothing diet mindset, and prevent you from feeling your best.

Advice: Try to strike a daily balance between enjoyable foods. As you go through the week, have a little serving of chocolate, chips, or your favorite snack food with your other meals and snacks.

5. Create a regular sleep schedule

There are a lot more factors influencing your eating choices than willpower. Insufficient sleep can heighten your appetite and increase the likelihood that you'll seek high-energy snack items like chips and cookies.

Advice: Establish a regular sleep schedule with a goal of 7-9 hours per night. Keep track of how your eating habits change the day after a sleepless night.

6. Put a high priority on food pleasure

Everybody wants to consume tasty meals. Therefore, if you're chowing down on tasteless chicken breast and dry salads in the name of losing weight, it won't be long until your appetites take control.

Advice: Include meals you usually appreciate in your healthy eating plan to increase satisfaction. You may enhance the taste of nutritious foods by including different textures, herbs, sauces, and dips.

7. Pay attention to stress management

Stress can disrupt your hunger and fullness cues, making it more difficult to eat consistently. It's also possible that you eat to deal with stress and other uncomfortable emotions, which can make eating consistently challenging.

Advice: Prioritize stress reduction in your daily activities. Examine techniques for managing emotions, such as counseling, social support, soothing baths, and mental health walks.

8. Ditch the "all or nothing" mentality

It's far too simple to fall into the trap of eating really "good" for a while and then really "bad." The goal of a sustained, healthful diet is to strike a balance between the two extremes.

Advice: Keep going even if you eat something decadent—or perhaps more than you intended to! Stop, think, and continue. Think about including some enjoyable items in your weekly meal plan.

9. A successful meal plan

Planning your meals entails knowing what to buy and how to prepare your food. And it becomes much easier to maintain your healthy diet throughout the hectic workweek as a result.

Advice: List the two to three meals and snacks you want to prepare this week and post them in your kitchen. If you're having trouble deciding what to make, look over this list.

10. Give up trying to exclude certain meals.

You wouldn't want to stick to a diet that forbids you from eating any of your favorite foods. A genuinely sustainable strategy will figure out how to incorporate your favorite foods into a well-balanced diet.

Advice: List five of your favorite meals and consider what you may add to make them more nourishing and full. For further balance, look for methods to incorporate fat, color, protein, or carbs.

It's not about perfection when it comes to eating consistently. Furthermore, if you've previously found it difficult to stick to diets, it's probably because they were excessively strict and unworkable.

FOOD RECIPES THAT SUPPORT GOOD GUT HEALTH

- ☐ Breakfasts
- ☐ Lunches
- ☐ Dinner
- ☐ Smoothies
- ☐ Teas

Prepare satisfying meals for yourself that promote a healthy digestive system. With at least 15 grams of protein per serving, these meals will help you support bone health, muscle repair, and safety. They also include prebiotic-rich meals including fruits, vegetables, nuts, seeds, and whole grains, as well as probiotic-rich foods like yogurt and kefir. By maintaining a healthy gut microbiome with a balanced diet, these foods can help reduce inflammation and the risk of chronic illnesses.

Breakfast Recipes

1. Breakfast platter with winter sunshine

This breakfast bowl recipe will help you reach your recommended intake of colorful fruits and vegetables and will also strengthen your immune system.

Ingredients:

- One cup of water
- A dash of salt
- 1/4 cup of traditional rolled oats
- ½ sliced tiny banana
- One tablespoon of hazelnut-chocolate spread
- A dab of brittle sea salt

Instructions:

In a small saucepan, bring water and a small pinch of normal salt to a boil.

After adding the oats, lower the heat to medium and cook, stirring now and again, for about five minutes, or until most of the liquid has been absorbed. After turning off the heat, cover and leave for two to three minutes. Add a banana, chocolate spread, and crumbly salt over top.

Oats that are branded as "gluten-free" should be consumed by those who have celiac disease or gluten sensitivity since oats can cross-contaminate with wheat and barley.

2. Recipe for Mushroom Omelet

Ingredients:

- A couple of tsp unsalted butter
- Two ounces of mixed sliced mushrooms, including shiitake, oyster, and cremini.
- One minced garlic clove
- Two big eggs
- One tablespoon of full-fat milk
- ½ teaspoon of freshly chopped tarragon
- One-half teaspoon of salt
- Half a teaspoon of crushed pepper
- Three tablespoons of fontina cheese, shredded
- ½ teaspoon of freshly chopped chives

Instructions:

In a small nonstick skillet set over medium heat, melt butter. Stir often and cook until the mushrooms are soft and have a light brown color, about 5 to 7 minutes.

Add the garlic and simmer, stirring frequently, for about one minute, or until fragrant.

Meanwhile, in a small bowl, whisk together the eggs, milk, tarragon, salt, and pepper. Stir the egg mixture into the pan and cook until the mushrooms are cooked. Cook until the egg forms a thin, even layer, rotating the pan to allow the egg to run over the sides.

Simmer for another one to two minutes, or until very little moist, lowering the heat if the food is browning too quickly. Add some cheese on top of it. Spoon onto a dish and garnish with chives.

3. Toast with sprouted grains, peanut butter, and banana

Ingredients:

- One piece of sprout-grain bread
- 1 tbsp peanut butter
- One medium banana, cut into slices
- Guidelines

Instructions:

Toast the bread. After spreading peanut butter on the toast, place slices of banana on top.

4. Raspberry Yogurt Cereal Bowl

Ingredients:

- One cup of plain yogurt without fat
- ½ cup little cereal with shredded wheat
- 1/4 cup of raw raspberries
- Two tsp little chocolate chips
- One tsp of pumpkin seeds
- One-half teaspoon of ground cinnamon

Instructions:

Add shredded wheat, raspberries, chocolate chips, pumpkin seeds, and cinnamon to the top of the yogurt in a bowl.

Sample our best-selling Chickpea & Quinoa Grain Bowl for a plant-based, high-protein lunchtime meal. Alternatively, stock up on our Best Chicken Salad for mouthwatering wraps, crackers, sandwiches, and more.

5. Probiotic-Rich Miso Cup Soup

Ingredients:

- One tablespoon of water
- Two tsp white miso
- Toasted sesame oil, one tsp
- One cup of brown rice, cooked
- One cup of frozen cooked, shelled edamame
- One tiny head of young bok choy cut thinly
- 3/4 cup of split, sliced scallions
- One box (7 ounces) of drained and cubed (1/2-inch) sesame-ginger baked tofu
- Lime juice, 1 1/2 tablespoons
- One and a half tsp freshly grated ginger
- Two and a quarter cups of low-sodium vegetable broth, split
- Serve with lime wedges (optional).

Instructions:

Mix the water, miso, and sesame oil in a small bowl and distribute the mixture among three 1-pint canning jars or microwaveable airtight containers (each containing approximately 2 tablespoons). Add 1/3 cup rice, 1/3 cup bok choy, 1/3 cup edamame, 1/4 cup scallions, 1/2 cup tofu, and 1/2 teaspoon each of lime juice and ginger on top of each. Refrigerate and cover for up to three days.

To make one soup jar: Fill the container with 3/4 cup of broth. Cover and microwave on High for 1-minute intervals, stirring in between, for 2 to 3 minutes total, or until the soup is boiling and the veggies are soft. Give it five minutes to cool. If preferred, garnish with a wedge of lime.

6. Avocados Stuffed with Salmon

Ingredients:

- Half a cup of low-fat Greek yogurt
- 1/4 cup finely chopped celery
- Two tablespoons of freshly chopped parsley
- One tablespoon of lime juice
- Two tsp of mayonnaise
- One tsp Dijon mustard
- One-half teaspoon of salt
- Half a teaspoon of crushed pepper
- Two five-ounce cans of drained, flaked, skin-and bone-free salmon
- Two avocados
- Chopped parsley as a garnish

Instructions:

In a medium bowl, thoroughly mix yogurt, celery, parsley, lime juice, mayonnaise, mustard, salt, and pepper. Mix thoroughly after adding the fish.

Cut avocados in half lengthwise, then remove the pits. Remove the flesh from each avocado half, reserving about 1 tablespoon for a small bowl. Using a fork, mash the avocado flesh that has been scooped out and add it to the salmon mixture.

Spoon approximately 1/4 cup of the salmon mixture into each half of the avocado and pile it on top. If you'd like, garnish with chives.

7. Hot Ramen Noodle Soup in a Cup

Ingredients:

- 1 ½ tablespoons vegetarian bouillon paste with reduced sodium
- 1/2 tsp white miso powder
- A half-teaspoon of garlic chili sauce
- 1/2 tsp finely chopped ginger
- ½ cup of carrot, shredded
- ¾ cup of shiitake mushrooms, sliced
- ½ cup finely chopped baby spinach
- Three halved hard-boiled eggs
- A quarter cup of cooked ramen noodles
- Three tablespoons of scallions cut.
- A spoonful of sesame seeds
- Three cups of extremely hot water, split

Instructions

Fill 3 pint-and-a-half-sized canning jars to the brim with the following contents: 1/2 tablespoon bouillon paste, teaspoon miso, teaspoon chili-garlic sauce, and teaspoon ginger.

In each jar, arrange 1/4 cup of carrot, 1/4 cup of mushrooms, 1/2 cup of spinach, 2 egg halves, and 1/2 cup of noodles. Add 1/4 teaspoon of sesame seeds and 1 tablespoon of onions to the top of each. Shut the jars.

Pour one cup of extremely hot water into one jar to produce one serving of noodles. Shut the container and give it a shake to blend. Cook, covered, on high for one minute at a time until very hot, around two to three minutes. Give it five minutes. Before consuming, stir.

8. Quinoa and Black Bean Bowl

Ingredients:

- ½ cup of rinsed canned black beans
- Half a cup of cooked quinoa
- Half a cup of hummus
- One tablespoon of lime juice
- ¼ medium-sized diced avocado
- three tsp of pico de gallo
- Two tablespoons of freshly cut cilantro

Instructions:

In a bowl, mix the quinoa and beans. In a small bowl, combine hummus and lime juice; thin with water to desired consistency. Add avocado, cilantro, and pico de gallo on top.

9. The Greatest Sandwich-Friendly Chicken Salad Recipe

Ingredients:

- One-half cup mayonnaise
- 1/4 cup Greek-style plain strained yogurt made with whole milk
- Two tsp lemon juice
- One tsp Dijon mustard
- One-fourth teaspoon of paprika
- One-fourth teaspoon of powdered garlic
- 1/4 tsp salt
- 1/4 tsp ground pepper
- 1/4 cup of finely chopped, freshly tender mixed herbs (such as chives, dill, and/or tarragon)
- Three cups of cooked chicken breast, finely shredded
- Half a cup of celery chopped finely
- 1/4 cup finely chopped shallot

Instructions:

In a sizable bowl, whisk together mayonnaise, yogurt, lemon juice, mustard, paprika, garlic powder, salt, and pepper until thoroughly blended and smooth. Add the herbs and stir. Stir until the chicken, celery, and shallot are well coated.

10. Red Beans and Rice with Chicken

Ingredients:

- Ten ounces of boneless, skinless chicken breasts divided into 1-inch halves
- One-half teaspoon each of salt and powdered black pepper
- One tablespoon of olive oil
- One medium-sized ¾ cup of finely chopped green sweet pepper
- One medium-sized diced onion, ½ cup
- Two minced garlic cloves and one (15-ounce) can without salt drained and washed the red beans.
- One ready-to-serve container of cooked brown rice, like the brand Minute ®
- ½ teaspoon of cumin powder
- One-third cup of low-sodium chicken broth and one-half teaspoon of cayenne
- Slices of lime

Directions:

1 sprinkle of cayenne pepper

Season chicken with black pepper and salt. When the chicken is no longer pink and the veggies are soft, add the chicken, sweet pepper, onion, and garlic. Cook and stir for 8 to 10 minutes.

Add the rice, beans, stock, cumin, and 1/4 teaspoon of cayenne pepper to the skillet with the chicken mixture. Warm up thoroughly. Accompany with wedges of lime. Feel free to add more cayenne pepper if preferred.

1. Wraps with Fish Tacos

Ingredients:

- One pound of skinless, 1/2–3/4-inch thick halibut filets, either fresh or frozen
- Nonstick cooking spray with olive oil
- One teaspoon of either regular or ancho chili powder
- 1/4 cup mildly soured cream
- ¼ cup of fruit salsa in the flavor you want
- Two cups of pre packaged coleslaw mix (shredded cabbage and carrot)
- 4 tacos made with whole-grain flour
- A single, 8.5-oz package of Colleen mix, or packaged shredded cabbage with carrot
- One wedge slice of lime

Instructions:

If the fish is frozen, thaw it. Warm up the broiler. Clean the fish and use paper towels to pat dry.

Measure the fish filets' thickness. Apply a thin layer of cooking spray on the unheated rack of a broiler pan fitted with foil. Fish should be placed on a rack. Add a dash of chili powder. When testing the fish with a fork, broil it 4 to 5 inches from the heat source for 4 to 6 minutes per 1/2-inch thickness, or until it flakes readily. Fish should be somewhat cooled. Fish should be flaked into bite-sized pieces using a fork.

Meanwhile, combine the 1/4 cup salsa and the sour cream in a medium-sized bowl. Toss to coat. Add the 2 cups of coleslaw mix. Spoon a mixture of cabbage over tortillas. Place fish on top. Tortillas should be rolled. Serve with extra cole slaw and lime wedges, if you'd like. Pass more salsa if you'd like.

2. Edamame and beet green salad

Ingredients:

- Two cups of mixed greens for salad
- One cup of shelled and thawed edamame and one medium raw beet, peeled and shredded (about half a cup)
- Two teaspoons of vinegar from red wine
- One tablespoon of freshly cut cilantro
- One tablespoon of pure olive oil
- One-half teaspoon of salt
- Freshly ground pepper according to taste

Instructions:

Put the edamame, beet, and greens on a big platter. In a small bowl, whisk together vinegar, oil, cilantro, salt, and pepper. One tablespoon of the dressing should be drizzled over the greens, then gently toss to coat. Pour the remaining dressing over the salad in its entirety.

Salad and dressing should be kept separately in the fridge for up to two days. Before adding the dressing to the salad, whisk it together.

3. Sandwich with avocado and white beans

Ingredients:

- Two medium avocados
- One fifteen-ounce bag of washed white beans
- Two tsp lemon juice
- One tablespoon of pure olive oil
- 1 grated garlic clove and ¼ teaspoon of freshly chopped thyme
- One-half teaspoon of ground pepper
- Eight pieces of toasted whole-wheat bread
- Eight thin, well-cut slices of Cheese with cheddar (about 4 ounces)
- Four cups of baby lettuce

Instructions:

In a medium bowl, mash together avocados, beans, lemon juice, oil, garlic, thyme, and pepper until well incorporated but with some chunks remaining. Divide evenly between 4 bread pieces (1/2 cup each).

Add 1/4 cup red peppers, 2 cheese pieces, 1 cup lettuce, and the remaining bread on top of each sandwich.

4. Lightly Dressed Chicken and Spinach with Creamy Feta

Ingredients:

- Delicious Feta Dressing
- One cup of feta cheese, crumbled
- 1/2 cup plain yogurt made with whole milk
- One tablespoon of pure olive oil
- One tablespoon of lemon juice
- Half a teaspoon of finely chopped garlic
- Half a teaspoon each of salt, pepper, and fresh dill; 1 1/2 tablespoons of chopped fresh dill salad
- One box (5 ounces) of baby spinach
- Two cups of cooked, shredded chicken breast
- One fifteen-ounce can of washed, salted chickpeas
- Two medium Persian cucumbers, cut into thin, angled slices

- One cup of bell peppers, sliced
- 1/4 cup of roasted almond slices (see Tip)

Instructions:

Get the dressing ready: In a small food processor, combine feta, yogurt, oil, lemon juice, garlic, salt, and pepper; process until smooth, about 10 seconds. Add dill and stir.

Get the salad ready: Arrange 4 plates with the spinach, chicken, chickpeas, cucumbers, peppers, and almonds on top. Before serving, drizzle each with 1/4 cup of dressing.

Before using nuts in a dish, toast them for the finest flavor. To toast the nuts, set them in a small dry skillet over medium-low heat and stir regularly for 2 to 4 minutes, or until aromatic.

For up to three days, refrigerate the dressing (Step 1) in an airtight container.

5. Hot Ramen Noodle Soup in Cups

Ingredients:

- 1 ½ tablespoons vegetarian bouillon paste with reduced sodium
- 1/2 tsp white miso powder
- A half-teaspoon of garlic chili sauce
- 1/2 tsp finely chopped ginger
- ½ cup of carrot, shredded
- ¾ cup of shiitake mushrooms, sliced
- ½ cup finely chopped baby spinach
- Three halved hard-boiled eggs
- A quarter cup of cooked ramen noodles
- Three tablespoons of scallions cut.
- A spoonful of sesame seeds
- Three cups of extremely hot water, split

Instructions

Fill Three pint-and-a-half-sized canning jars with 1/2 tablespoon bouillon paste, and 1/2 teaspoon with miso, 1/2 teaspoon with chili-garlic sauce, and 1/2 teaspoon with ginger.

In each jar, arrange 1/4 cup of carrot, 1/4 cup of mushrooms, 1/2 cup of spinach, 2 egg halves, and 1/2 cup of noodles. Add 1/4 teaspoon of sesame seeds and 1 tablespoon of onions to the top of each. Shut the jars.

Pour one cup of extremely hot water into one jar to produce one serving of noodles. Shut the container and give it a shake to blend. Cook, covered, on high for one minute at a time until very hot, around two to three minutes. Give it five minutes. Before consuming, stir.

To prepare ahead of time: Covered precooked jars can be kept in the fridge for up to three days.

Dinner Recipes

1. Dinner broccolini with Garlic-Anchovy Pasta

Ingredients:

- Two tablespoons of pure olive oil
- 6 filets of anchovies (see Tip)
- Four garlic cloves, cut thinly
- A dash of crushed red pepper
- One box (5 ounces) of baby spinach
- Angel hair pasta made with whole wheat, 8 ounces
- One bunch of broccoli rabe or two bunches of broccolini, cut coarsely and trimmed
- ¼ cup of freshly chopped parsley
- ¼ teaspoon salt and ½ cup chopped, roasted almonds
- Four ounces of crumbled goat cheese
- Grated zest of lemon as a garnish

Instructions:

Warm up some oil in a big skillet over medium heat. Add the anchovies, garlic, and crushed red pepper. Cook for two minutes, or until the anchovies become fragrant, pushing them up with the back of a wooden spoon. Cook the spinach for approximately a minute, stirring periodically, in two batches until it has barely wilted. To stay warm, remove from the heat and cover.

Boil the water, add the pasta and broccolini (or broccoli rabe), and simmer for 3 to 5 minutes, or until the pasta is just soft. Set aside one cup of the cooking liquid. After draining, add the pasta and veggies to the skillet and toss to mix, adding just enough of the set-aside water to get the right consistency. Toss with salt and parsley, then top with goat cheese and almonds for serving. If desired, garnish with lemon zest.

Anchovies, a tiny fish with a big taste, add a ton of umami to this pasta. For the most environmentally friendly choice, look for packages bearing the blue Marine Stewardship Council certification logo.

2. Sun-Dried Tomato & White Bean Gnocchi

Ingredients:

- ½ cup of sliced sun-dried tomatoes packed with oil and two tablespoons of jarred oil, split
- One (16-oz) pack of gnocchi that is shelf-stable
- One fifteen-ounce can of rinsed low-sodium cannellini beans
- One box (5 ounces) of baby spinach
- One big chopped shallot
- ⅓ cup low-sodium chicken broth or broth without chicken.
- One-third cup of heavy cream
- One tablespoon of lemon juice
- Three teaspoons of recently picked basil

Instructions:

In a big nonstick skillet, heat 1 tablespoon of oil over medium-high heat. Add gnocchi and simmer, tossing frequently, for about 5 minutes, or until plumped and beginning to brown. After adding the beans and spinach, simmer for one minute, or until the spinach has wilted. Move to a platter.

Transfer the leftover tablespoon of oil into the pan and set it on medium heat. Stir in shallot and sun-dried tomatoes and simmer for 1 minute. Simmer for about two minutes, or until the liquid has mostly evaporated.

Whisk in the cream, lemon juice, salt, and pepper after lowering the heat to medium. Pour the sauce back over the gnocchi mixture by stirring it in. Garnish with basil and serve.

3. Cheesy Pizzas with Cauliflower Steak

Ingredients:

- One packet (9 ounces) of fresh spinach spaghetti
- One tablespoon of pure olive oil
- 4 ounces diced pancetta
- One sixteen-ounce container of thawed frozen baby lima beans
- 1 cup of shallots, sliced
- Two minced garlic cloves
- One-half teaspoon of dehydrated rosemary
- Four cups of baby spinach
- Three tsp lemon juice
- ¾ cup of finely shredded pecorino cheese, split

Instructions:

After adding the pasta, cook it according to the directions on the package. First, drain the pasta and set aside a cup of water.

Heat a large skillet with oil over medium-high heat in the meantime. When crispy, add the pancetta and cook, turning occasionally, for 6 to 8 minutes. Slotted spoon for transferring to a plate. The pan should now contain shallots and lima beans. Reduce heat and simmer until the shallots are tender, stirring occasionally, about 3 minutes. When aromatic, stir-fry the garlic and rosemary for about one minute after adding them. Add the spinach and cook until it wilts about 2 minutes.

To the pan, add the pasta and the water that was set aside. Cook for approximately a minute, stirring occasionally, or until the sauce thickens. Add half of the pecorino, the pancetta, and lemon juice. Top the spaghetti with the remaining pecorino cheese and serve.

4. Cheesy Pizzas with Cauliflower Steak

Ingredients:

- Two cups of finely chopped green cabbage
- Two tablespoons of freshly cut cilantro
- Lime juice, two tablespoons
- One-half teaspoon of salt
- Half an avocado, mashed
- Half a jalapeño-cheddar bagel toasted
- One cup of cooked, rinsed, canned black beans without salt

Instructions:

In a medium bowl, toss together cabbage, cilantro, lime juice, and salt. Top each half of a bagel with a spread of avocado. Place half the slaw and 1/2 cup of beans on top of each.

5. Curry with Vegan Coconut Chickpeas

Ingredients:

- Two teaspoons of canola or avocado oil
- One cup of finely chopped onion
- One cup of bell peppers, chopped
- One medium zucchini, chopped into halves.
- One fifteen-ounce can of rinsed and drained chickpeas
- 1 ½ cups simmer sauce with coconut curry (see Tip)
- 1/4 cup veggie broth and 4 cups baby spinach
- Two cups of brown rice that has already been cooked; reheat per package directions.

Instructions:

Add the onion, pepper, and zucchini. Cook for 5 to 6 minutes, turning frequently, or until the vegetables start to brown.

Stir the sauce and broth till they simmer and stir in the chickpeas. Simmer the vegetables for four to six minutes, or until they are soft, on medium-low heat. Just before serving, stir in the spinach. Put it on top of rice.

6. Pita, Hummus, and Tabbouleh Plate

Ingredients:

- Double-cup tabbouleh (see Tips)
- One cup beet hummus (see Tips)
- One cup of sugar snap peas cut off the stems of four radishes
- One cup of mixed olives
- One cup of raspberries
- One cup of blackberries
- Four whole-wheat pita breads (4 inches)
- ⅔ cup dry-roasted, unsalted pistachios
- 4 cookie vegans (see Tips)

Instructions:

Divide the contents among 4 plates equally.

Make prepared tabbouleh, the well-known whole-grain salad from the Middle East, for

convenience, but make our delicious, fresh-tasting Parsley Tabbouleh recipe if you have the time.

Try our Roasted Beet Hummus recipe if your local grocery store doesn't have beet hummus.

Use the Vegan No-Bake Cookies recipe from EatingWell or pack your favorite vegan cookies.

To prepare ahead, divide the ingredients into individual table containers.

7. Black bean vegan burgers

Ingredients:

- One 15.5-oz can of washed, unsalted black beans
- One cup of cooked quinoa
- ½ cup panko breadcrumbs made entirely of wheat
- ½ cup finely sliced onions
- One spoonful of tomato paste without additional salt
- 1 ½ tablespoons of cumin powder
- ½ teaspoon powdered chipotle chiles
- One-half teaspoon of powdered garlic
- Divide a half-cup of vegan mayonnaise.
- Split a ½ teaspoon of salt.
- One medium avocado
- Lime juice, two tablespoons
- Two tablespoons of freshly cut cilantro
- Two tsp water
- Two tablespoons of pure olive oil
- Six tiny toasted whole-wheat hamburger buns

- Six tiny tomato slices

Instructions:

With your hands, mash together the beans, quinoa, panko, scallions, tomato paste, cumin, chili powder, garlic powder, 1/4 cup mayonnaise, and 1/4 teaspoon salt in a large bowl. Form into six patties that are 3/4 inch thick. Place the patties onto a plate and chill for 10 minutes. In a food processor, combine avocado, water, lime juice, cilantro, the remaining 1/4 cup mayonnaise, and 1/4 teaspoon salt; process until smooth, about 30 seconds.

In a large cast-iron skillet, heat the oil over medium-high heat. Add the patties and cook for 3 to 4 minutes on each side or until golden brown. Split the avocado mixture equally between the top and bottom sides of the buns. Place the tomato slices and bean patties equally between the bottom and top bread halves.

8. Chickpeas atop romaine lettuce

Ingredients:

- Clothes
- One pitted and peeled avocado
- A half-cup of buttermilk
- ¼ cup finely chopped fresh herbs, like cilantro, mint, sorrel, parsley, or tarragon
- Two tsp of rice vinegar
- Half a teaspoon of salt
- Lettuce
- Chopped romaine lettuce, three cups
- One cup of cucumbers, sliced
- One fifteen-ounce can of washed chickpeas
- ¼ cup of low-fat Swiss cheese, chopped
- Half the six cherry tomatoes, if preferred

Instructions:

In a blender, combine the avocado, buttermilk, herbs, vinegar, and salt to make the dressing. Blend until smooth.

To make the salad, combine the cucumber and lettuce with 1/4 cup of the dressing in a bowl. Add tomatoes, cheese, and chickpeas on top. (Keep the extra dressing chilled for up to three days.)

Make ahead: Store any leftover dressing in the refrigerator covered for up to three days.

9. Well-Composed Bean Salad with Basil Dressing

Instructions:

- Two cups of cut green beans, or around eight ounces
- Add ½ cup chopped fresh basil and 2 teaspoons chopped for decoration.
- One little shallot, cut into quarters
- Half a cup of extra virgin olive oil.
- Three tsp red wine vinegar
- Two tsp honey or syrup made from agave
- Two tsp Dijon mustard
- One-half teaspoon of salt
- One-half teaspoon of ground pepper
- One fifteen-ounce can (see tip) of washed chickpeas
- One fifteen-oz can of washed dark red kidney beans
- One 15-oz can of rinsed black beans

- One fifteen-ounce can of washed cannellini or navy beans
- 1 cup of cherry tomatoes, divided into 2
- ½ cup of radishes, cut very thinly

Instructions

Put green beans in a big pot with a steamer basket on it and steam for about 4 minutes, or until they are crisp-tender. To cool them, spread them out.

In the meantime, blend 1/2 cup basil, shallot, oil, vinegar, mustard, honey (or agave), salt, and pepper in a blender. Blend until smooth.

Place the green beans and all the other ingredients onto a serving dish. Accompany the dish with the dressing. If preferred, garnish with the chopped basil.

Preparation Tip: Keep the dressing (Step 2) and green beans (Step 1) separate and covered in the refrigerator for up to a day.

Do not use canned beans; try making your own. Rinse well and start with 1 pound of dry beans of any kind. Transfer to a sizable bowl and add two inches of cold water to cover. Soak overnight for at least eight hours.

(If you need to cook the beans quickly, place them in a pot with two inches of water, bring to a boil, boil for two minutes, then take the pot off the heat and leave it covered for an hour.) After the beans are drained, add them to a big saucepan, and cover them with three inches of cold water. Skim off any foam as you bring it to a boil. Lower the heat to a low simmer and let the beans cook, stirring from time to time, for 30 to 2 hours, or until they are soft. (Cooking times vary according to bean type and age; begin testing for tenderness at 30 minutes.)

Add salt only when beans are almost ready; adding salt too soon will keep the beans from softening. Beans can be frozen for up to three months or refrigerated in their cooking liquid for up to one week (use around one teaspoon of salt per pound of beans). Dry beans yield five to six cups per pound.

10. Quinoa with Chipotle Burrito Bowl

Ingredients:

- 1 tablespoon of chipotle chiles in adobo sauce, finely chopped.
- One tablespoon of pure olive oil
- One-half teaspoon of powdered garlic
- ½ teaspoon of cumin powder
- One-pound chicken breast, deboned and skinless
- One-half teaspoon of salt
- Two cups of quinoa, cooked
- Two cups of romaine lettuce, shredded
- One cup of rinsed canned pinto beans
- One diced ripe avocado
- ¼ cup of ready-made salsa, such as pico de gallo
- Half a cup of shredded Monterey Jack or Cheddar cheese
- Slices of lime for serving

Instructions:

Set the broiler to average or high heat.

In a small bowl, mix chipotle, oil, cumin, and garlic powder.

If broiling, oil a rimmed baking sheet or the grill rack (see Tip). Add salt to the chicken to season it. On the baking sheet that has been prepared, broil or grill the chicken for five or nine minutes. After flipping, brush with the chipotle glaze, and cook for a further 3 to 5 minutes on the grill or 9 minutes under the broiler, or until an instant-read thermometer inserted in the thickest section registers 165 degrees F. Move to a sanitized chopping board. Dice into little pieces.

Add 1/2 cup quinoa, 1/2 cup chicken, 1/2 cup lettuce, 1/4 cup beans, 1/4 avocado, 1 tablespoon cheese, and 1 tablespoon pico de gallo (or other salsa) to each burrito bowl. Garnish with a wedge of lime.

Using tongs, coat a folded paper towel with oil, then rub the oily surface all over the grill rack. (Using cooking spray on a hot grill is not advised.)

Smoothie Recipes

1. Smoothie with spinach, peanut butter, and bananas

Ingredients:

- One cup of plain kefir
- One tablespoon of peanut butter
- One cup of spinach
- One banana, frozen
- One tablespoon honey, if desired

Instructions:

In a blender, combine the kefir, peanut butter, spinach, banana, and honey (if desired). Process till smooth.

2. Kefir and Berry Smoothie

Ingredients:

- A quarter-cup of frozen mixed berries
- One cup of plain kefir
- Half a medium banana
- Two tsp of almond butter
- One-half teaspoon of vanilla extract

Instructions:

Blend banana, kefir, peanut butter, raspberries, and flax meal in a blender. Blend until smooth, adding a spoonful of water at a time as needed.

3. Banana & Almond Butter Protein Smoothie

Ingredients:

- One tiny frozen banana
- 1 cup almond milk without sugar
- Two tsp almond butter
- Two tablespoons of protein powder without flavor
- One tablespoon of your preferred sweetener (optional)
- One-half teaspoon of ground cinnamon
- Four to six ice cubes

Ingredients:

In a blender, blend all the ingredients till smooth.

4. Avocado yogurt mix

Ingredients:

- One cup of plain yogurt without fat
- One cup of raw spinach
- One banana, frozen
- Half an avocado
- Two tsp water
- One tsp honey

Instructions:

In a blender, combine yogurt, spinach, banana, avocado, water, and honey. Blend until smooth.

5. Banana-Cocoa Soy Smoothie

Ingredients:

- One banana
- One-third cup of silken tofu
- Half a cup of soy milk
- Two tsp of cocoa powder without sugar added
- One tablespoon of honey

Instructions:

Banana slices should be frozen until solid. In a blender, whisk together tofu, soymilk, chocolate, and honey until smooth. After adding the banana slices through the lid's opening while the motor is running, blend the mixture until it is smooth.

Tea Recipes

A calming cup of herbal tea after a meal is a kinder and more pleasurable cure than over-the-counter medications when you are experiencing digestive problems or stomach troubles.

A healthy gut can be naturally supported by using herbs. Many have been used for thousands of years to cure digestive problems, ranging from nausea and diarrhea to constipation and bloating. Furthermore, there's growing scientific proof that these home treatments work wonders for digestive problems.

A tasty approach to increase the amount of herbs in your diet is through herbal teas. They also assist you in meeting your daily water intake targets. Drinking plenty of fluids is important when you are having digestive problems because dehydration can lead to these problems.

These are the top seven herbal teas that promote gut health and digestion.

1. Tea Peppermint

Any dinner is better finished with a cup of peppermint tea. It is also very beneficial to the health of your digestive system. It should come as no surprise that peppermint has been used since the Ancient Egyptians to treat dyspepsia.

Menthol is a chemical found in peppermint. This active component appears to be the reason peppermint tea works so well as a digestive aid. Abdominal pain and other symptoms linked to irritable bowel syndrome (IBS) can be lessened by peppermint.

In addition to preventing indigestion and nausea, peppermint calms the colon and esophagus.

One of our best-selling flagship teas has raspberry leaves and peppermint in it. Excellent for individuals who are pregnant or experiencing menstruation difficulties, this tea is also a fantastic option for those who have digestive problems.

2. Ginger Tea

An essential plant in Ayurveda, the age-old, holistic Indian medical system, is fiery ginger. This is because Ayurvedic therapy places a lot of emphasis on the gut to maintain the health and strength of the digestive fire or agni.

There are many digestive benefits associated with ginger. It helps reduce nausea and stop vomiting during the first trimester of pregnancy when it is frequently given. However, you don't need to be pregnant to benefit from ginger. It relieves a variety of stomach discomforts, such as motion sickness, indigestion, and chemotherapy-induced nausea.

Because of its flavor and health advantages, ginger is a staple in many of our tea blends. Ginger is combined with other beneficial herbs in our NutraCleanse and NutraTrim teas to improve digestive health. You might also sample our trademark tea, Ginger & Ginseng.

3. Fennel Tea

Among its many benefits is its ability to relieve digestive issues. Due to its antibacterial and anti-inflammatory properties, fennel tea promotes good digestion and helps rebalance the gut.

Fennel works well against a variety of bad germs, including those that give rise to gastrointestinal problems like indigestion and diarrhea. Additionally, it lessens IBS symptoms including stomach pain.

Another reason we like to use fennel in a lot of our teas is that it gives a beautiful taste to any herbal tea blend. It's a key component of our NutraTrim tea, which we blend with other herbs to support digestive health and reduce appetite.

4. Dandelion root tea

Though its cheery yellow blooms are their most well-known feature, dandelions' roots are used as a traditional herbal cure for a variety of ailments, including stomach problems.

The active ingredients in dandelion root facilitate the passage of food through our digestive tracts, thus supporting a healthy digestive system. Dandelion root, being an abundant antioxidant, also aids in the fight against inflammation, which is frequently the root cause of digestive problems.

A nice tea to try if you are feeling bloated is dandelion root. Since it works as an effective diuretic, it can reduce bloating and water retention.

To improve kidney function, boost digestion, and assist your liver in eliminating toxins, we add dandelion root to our NutraCleanse tea. It is also an essential component of our teas, NutraTrim and NutraRelease.

5. Artichoke tea

It is common knowledge that artichokes assist our livers and aid in our detoxification following a period of excess. It also provides additional health benefits, particularly for digestion.

One kind of prebiotic fiber found in artichokes is called inulin. Prebiotics are a source of nourishment for the healthy bacteria that are already present in our guts, as opposed to probiotics, which contain the beneficial bacteria that our digestive systems require. This maintains our digestive systems functioning properly and aids in maintaining a healthy balance.

Regular use of artichoke extract also contributes to an increase in the number of good bacteria in the stomach.

Artichokes are used in our NutraCleanse tea to promote healthy digestion and liver function.

6. Licorice tea

Naturally sweet Licorice tastes great added to any herbal tea. It has been used for ages as a herbal treatment and also supports the health of your intestines.

Liquorice, like artichokes, is excellent in shielding your liver and maintaining its proper function in ridding your body of toxins. In addition to being a useful treatment for indigestion, licorice also eases acid reflux and heartburn.

Our signature tea, made with licorice and cinnamon, is a delightfully warming blend that is both energizing and grounding. Additionally, we utilize licorice in our NutraCleanse tea blend, along with other digestive-supporting herbs.

7. Winter tea

Turmeric is another herb for herbal tea that we suggest for anyone who wants to keep their digestive system in good working order because of its anti-inflammatory qualities.

Turmeric is one of the main herbs used in Ayurveda, along with ginger. Western medicine is beginning to recognize the advantages of this potent component as well.

Curcumin is the primary active ingredient in turmeric. This antioxidant has the potential to alleviate symptoms associated with a variety of digestive disorders, such as colitis and irritable bowel syndrome.

Turmeric supplements can help us digest food more easily and prevent digestive problems by enhancing the flora in our stomachs.

We've blended cinnamon and turmeric to create one of our favorite comforting signature teas.

8. Debloat Tea

This particular tea helped me alot with my bloat, and all the ingredients are regular herbs we use in our kitchen. I take it first thing in the morning when I wake up on an empty stomach.

Ingredient:

- Lemon
- Turmeric
- Ginger
- Apple cider vinegar

Instructions:

Wash the ginger and turmeric properly and you can either peel the bark or blend it like that, they should be equal in proportions, then squeeze in some lemon, about ½ to 1 cup depending on the amount of ginger and turmeric you are blending.

Add the same amount of apple cider vinegar, and boil on very low heat for 2 minutes, strain out the liquid and you can put this into the freezer and add warm water anytime you want to take it in the morning.

9. Constipation Relief Tea

This is saved for last, as it is very unorthodox. So, this should be your very last resort.

Remember we talked about gut - brain connection? Well, your body can get used to your routine of not pooping in weeks and even when you have done everything right, the mind would still need to be encouraged to remember to send signals for bowel movement.

So, you can encourage this behavior by using this tea.

Ingredients

- Cascara sagrada herb
- Licorice

Instructions:

Boil over low heat for 5 minutes and strain the liquid. The liquid should be taken before bed.

Remember, your body should not need medicine to function, it should need just food, do not abuse any of these teas, take as infrequently as possible.

Conclusions

I know for a fact, that the information in this book will help you and more importantly, give you a permanent solution to all your gut health problems.

Sometimes, for the most complex problems, the simpler the solution.

I look forward to hearing about how the contents in this book shapes your health and overall well being in the coming weeks, as you apply them without fail.

I would like to implore you to kindly take out a few minutes of your time, to let me know what you genuinely think of the information in this book, your review will help many others out there solve their gut health problems too.